Intermittent Fasting

Beginners Guide to Intermittent Fasting For Weight Loss!

Table of Contents

Introduction

In case you have already heard of intermittent fasting, but don't know how it works, this is the perfect book for you. During the course of this book, you will learn how Intermittent Fasting works, how beneficial it is and to make it simple for you. Many consider the idea of intermittent fasting as a difficult task or an unsafe method, which could cause complications to their health. Though there are side effects associated with this method, it gets serious only when the person using this type of fast is not careful about choosing his diet protocol. Therefore, it is crucial to understand Intermittent Fasting before you practice it.

Intermittent fasting is simple when compared to other fasting methods. You need to fast for the prescribed period of time, and then consume the calories required for your body during the eating window. This eating window can be for six to eight hours on an average in a day. Does it sound unhealthy or uncomfortable to you? Well, it isn't. This fasting method is a useful tool to improve your dietary compliance. Many people who had already practiced intermittent fasting enjoy the method more than the traditional eating patterns people use in this day and age. This is because it allows you to have larger meals during the eating window.

Have you been struggling to lose weight for a long time? Then this book has the perfect solution for you. Intermittent fasting can help you lose weight by getting rid of that extra fat and flab on your body. You need to ensure you fit this fasting method into your regular routine in the right way. Choose a well-balanced approach that will work best for your body type, lifestyle and health goals.

It is crucial to know how to make intermittent fasting work best for your body. You should be able to get your work style, daily routine and eating habits in place. It can be pretty tricky to follow the fasting method due to the following criteria:

> Your exercise routine
> Your meal time
> Your work routine, etc

While intermittent fasting, you need to make exercise a priority and, at the same time, eat better.

In this book, we will discuss what intermittent fasting is, its role to help lose weight and the various other benefits it provides. It is essential to enjoy the positive aspects of this diet, as it is good for your mind and body. The chapters in this book will help you understand more about intermittent fasting, the various fasting methods and the ways to get started. The chapters will also talk about how to boost your immune system and increase longevity.

I hope this book serves as an informative and interesting! Please sign up to our page by followig this link: http://eepurl.com/dv48LX.

Happy Reading!

the solitary and utter responsibility of the recipient reader. Under no circumstances will any legal responsibility or blame be held against the publisher for any reparation, damages, or monetary loss due to the information herein, either directly or indirectly.

Respective authors own all copyrights not held by the publisher.

The information herein is offered for informational purposes solely, and is universal as so. The presentation of the information is without contract or any type of guarantee assurance.

The trademarks that are used are without any consent, and the publication of the trademark is without permission or backing by the trademark owner. All trademarks and brands within this book are for clarifying purposes only and are the owned by the owners themselves, not affiliated with this document.

Chapter 1 What is Intermittent Fasting?

So what exactly is intermittent fasting and why does it work? Intermittent Fasting (IF) may just be the best-kept secret of the diet and fitness industry. With over 100 years of research to back up this amazing game changing lifestyle, intermittent fasting is poised to take the health and wellness community by storm.

Before we jump into what intermittent fasting is, and why it works, let's first go over a couple of things that intermittent fasting is not.

First, intermittent fasting is NOT a diet plan. There are no off-limits foods, no meal plans, no meal prepping, and no complicated recipes. In fact, you can practice intermittent fasting and eat whatever you want. You'll still get some of the benefits. Of course, intermittent fasting works the best when you try to eat more vegetables and whole foods, while eating less processed foods. It isn't necessary, and you can keep having treats without any guilt.

Second, intermittent fasting is NOT a metabolism lowering calorie restriction game. In fact, intermittent fasting can be used to lose weight, maintain weight, or even gain muscle. What does this mean for you? If you like intermittent fasting, and it ends up being a good fit, you can practice it for the rest of your life. It helps you lose weight, of course, but it has so many more benefits than just that.

How Does Intermittent Fasting Work?

If you want to know what makes intermittent fasting help you burn fat, you initially need to comprehend the distinction between the fasted state and the fed state.

When your body is processing and retaining nourishment, it is considered fed state. Normally, this state begins when you start eating and goes on for three to five hours while your body processes and ingests the sustenance you just consumed. In the fed state your insulin levels are high and so your body finds it difficult to burn up fat.

Once this time period is over, the next state is the post-absorptive state during which your body isn't digesting or processing food. The post–absorptive state continues up to 12 hours after your last food intake, which is the point at which your body enters the fasted state. Your body finds it much easier to burn fat in this state thanks to its lower insulin levels.

In the fasted state, your body can actually consume fat that it didn't have access to while it was in the fed state. Since our bodies don't enter the fasted state for at least 8 hours after the last meal we consumed, they are rarely in the state that allows them to burn fat. It is no wonder then that those people who take up intermittent fasting find that they are losing fat without making any significant changes to what they consume, how much of it they consume or how much they work out. Thanks to fasting, your body goes into a state of fat consumption that it is rarely able to do when you're eating normally.

Fasting for brief periods enables individuals to eat less calories, and furthermore streamlines a few hormones identified with weight control.

There are a few diverse intermittent fasting methods. Three well known ones are:

The 16/8 Method: Skip breakfast each day and eat amid a 8-hour eating window, for example, from 12 twelve to 8 pm.

Eat-Stop-Eat: Do maybe a couple 24-hour fasts every week, for instance by not having from supper one day until supper the following day.

The 5:2 Diet: Only eat 500-600 calories on two days of the week, yet eat ordinarily the other 5 days.

For whatever length of time that you don't try to make up for it by eating significantly more amid the non-fasting periods, at that point these methods will prompt lessened calorie admission and enable you to get in shape and lose tummy fat.

Chapter 2 How To Get Started In Intermittent Fasting

While intermittent fasting is pretty simple to follow, the information here will greatly make it even easier for you to get started and succeed while at it.

1.Begin with one day

Like anything new in life, if you want to set yourself up for success, it is very important to start small with intermittent fasting. So what exactly does starting small mean with regards to intermittent fasting?

Well, you can start by pushing your meals a little so that you take longer to take the next meal then over time, you can get to a point where you can actually skip an entire meal. For instance, instead of taking breakfast at 7-8am, you can push it by about 1 hour to 1 hour 30 minutes to eat between 8 and 9.30 am. You could then not take lunch at 1pm and instead push it to 4 or 5 pm. If you eat this late, you could comfortably take a smaller meal for dinner or skip the meal altogether. This will get you accustomed to taking more time between meals, which will ultimately help you to at fast for at least 16 hours comfortably. Over time, you can then increase the duration of your fasting window to ultimately get to 24-48 hours if you are up to it.

In case you find intermittent fasting tough, adopting creatine monohydrate can help provide the body with enough energy to carry out metabolic functions.

2. Determine your goals

Before you choose a suitable intermittent fasting protocol, you need to determine your goals. For instance, if you want to boost your body composition in terms of fat loss or growth of muscles, 16 hours of fast with 8 hours of feeding window practiced everyday can work for you. To facilitate body cleansing and to prevent aging, a 36 hours period of fasting is recommended provided don't go past 72 hours.

3. Time the fasting for social purposes

For beginners, it's easier to set your 8 hours intermittent fasting window anywhere between 9.30 in the morning and around 5.30 in the evening especially while in social places. However, having such a "social" program helps you eat more meals and calories, which technically means you may cheat more often. Furthermore, you may still get tempted to eat even after 5.30pm or soon after you leave job. The effective approach to avoid cheating too often is to skip breakfast and midmorning snack then eat your meals between 12 noon and 8pm.

4. Take water for breakfast

You can decide to fast overnight until 12 noon and so taking water in the morning is a good strategy to keep hunger at bay during breakfast. Consider drinking 1-2 glasses of water after waking up to help revitalize the body previously dehydrated during your sleep. To ensure that you "enjoy" water as your regular breakfast drink, add lemon flavoring as lime or lemon juice helps add favor and pleasant smell to ordinary water.

5. Choose tea or coffee

In addition to water, taking tea or coffee is a great idea provided that you don't add sweeteners such as sugar or cream. Aim to drink the tea or Bulletproof® coffee warm to fight most hunger pangs. The Bulletproof® coffee is enriched with butter and MCT oil, which provides calories required by the body to do mandatory cellular functions such as cell repair.

6. Have a day to indulge

While having a "cheat day" helps you stick to the fasting program primarily because you'll indulge in whatever foods you like, you can control such eating by choosing healthier ingredients. Have a few high calorie days where you focus on unprocessed and natural foods such as sweet potatoes, almond butter, 85% dark chocolate etc. Do not just indulge on sweet foods as you might reverse all gains you make in terms of weight loss.

Chapter 3 The Health Benefits Of Intermittent Fasting

Intermittent fasting has helped many people lose weight and become the best versions of them. This pattern of eating is not a short-term diet, but a long-term lifestyle. Why? Because it has a whole list of research backed health benefits that go way beyond weight loss.

Do you have complicated medical histories in your family? Maybe you're nervous about diabetes, or heart disease. The fact is, when the body is in fasting mode, you release hormones that tell the cells in your body that it is time to go into repair mode. In this repair mode, the cells can eliminate many of the first signs of disease. By practicing intermittent fasting, we give our cells more time to heal, providing ourselves with increased longevity in our lives.

Intermittent Fasting and Diabetes

The first health benefit to come from intermittent fasting originates with that little, fat regulating chemical, insulin. Insulin is probably the most famous for its role in causing or preventing the onset of diabetes.

Today, diabetes is not a debilitating disease, as long as it is caught early and dealt with responsibly. As a matter of fact, most people don't need to suffer from diabetes. Adding intermittent fasting to your lifestyle can help prevent the onset of type 2 diabetes.

Type 2 diabetes is the form of the disease that is mostly triggered by an unhealthy diet and lifestyle. The body develops insulin resistance and therefore cannot regulate the amount of sugar in the blood stream.

When we practice intermittent fasting, the body lowers its overall insulin level. Periods of low insulin help us prevent against insulin resistance. In one study conducted on human subjects, blood sugar was reduced up to 6% during a fast. During that same fast, the insulin level in the body was reduced from 20 to 31%!

A further study conducted in rats with diabetes showed that intermittent fasting helped prevent and protect the kidney from damage. This has not yet been tested in humans.

Okay, so intermittent fasting helps prevent diabetes. But what if diabetes isn't a concern for you? No one in your family has ever had diabetes and your diet right now isn't that bad. Okay, fine. What about a much more common and more deadly disease? What about cancer?

Intermittent Fasting and Cancer

It's true, intermittent fasting can help prevent and protect the body from developing certain cancers. How? Let's find out.

First, intermittent fasting can reduce oxidative stress and inflammation in the body. Oxidative stress is a fancy way of talking about the cell's natural ability to detoxify itself. If this process of detoxification is interrupted or blocked, oxidative stress occurs. Unfortunately, eating a bad diet, or overeating, can lead to increased oxidative stress and inflammation in the body. These two things can lead to cancer.

There have been a few studies that illustrate the relationship between intermittent fasting and reduced oxidative stress and inflammation. If you're trying to prevent or even heal a chronic disease, or cancer, intermittent fasting could be an excellent choice for you.

Okay, but what if you, or someone you love, already has cancer? Based on a study done on human patients, there is some evidence that intermittent fasting can help reduce some of the side effects of chemotherapy!

Probably the most important benefit of intermittent fasting is it's ability to trigger autophagy in the cells. What is autophagy? It's a fancy way of saying "repair mode". When we are eating every three hours, cells are constantly reproducing, using the new food to create new cells. Yet when we pause and enter a short fasting period, the cells shift into repair mode.

This repair mode, known as autophagy, is essential for health cellular life in our bodies. Increasing the amount of repair in our bodies can protect us against certain diseases, including cancer, and Alzheimer's.

Intermittent Fasting and The Brain

Yes, that's right, IF can even help prevent Alzheimer's. The research on this claim is still rudimentary, but preliminary studies on rats show that intermittent fasting may delay or slow the onset of Alzheimer's. We need more research on human studies before we can make any bolder claims than that, but for now, better safe than sorry, right?

Even if Alzheimer's isn't a concern for you, there are many more benefits to the brain from intermittent fasting. The boost that IF gives to your metabolism also impacts your brain function.

Studies in animals have shown that intermittent fasting reduces brain damage, strokes, and improves mental functioning over time. Maybe eating your Wheaties in the morning isn't so important, after all.

Intermittent Fasting and The Heart

You may think we are done here. There can't be ANY more health benefits, right? Wrong. There is one more major health benefit to be earned from a lifestyle of intermittent fasting: lowered risk of heart disease.

Today in America, heart disease is a killer. It is one of the leading causes of death among adults, especially among adults struggling with obesity or weight gain.

Good news for American adults. Intermittent fasting has been shown, through animal studies, to improve on many different risk factors related to heart disease. It reduces blood pressure, cholesterol levels, blood triglycerides, inflammation, and blood sugar levels. Really, there can't be a better lifestyle choice out there where heart health is concerned.

Chapter 4 Fasting for Weight Loss

Dieting for a long time to get a short-term result really is not worth it. No matter the kind of diet you have been placed on, whether it is a low-calorie diet, the Atkins diet, or the low-fat diet of the Mediterranean model, they all unfortunately produce short-term results. It will take little or no time before you start regaining the weight you have just lost. Even the low carb diets that have proven effective over time are only good for short-term results, until there is regain of weight. This is commonly known as the "Jo-Jo-Effect". You should really ask why it is always like this. Continuously complying with dietary guides without laid out strategies will only yield a futile endeavour in the long run. The phrase "Eat less, Move more" is not as effective as it sounds.

You probably might have heard people saying, "The proof is in the pudding", which actually used to be "The proof of the pudding is in the eating". What does that even mean? It is important that you check the end results of anything you are doing before concluding if it is successful or not. You might have a notion that it will work, but that does not really mean it will.

Applying this to the popular disease obesity: for many years now, all we have been hearing and reading in health magazines has been "calories out, calories in". What this simply means is that taking lesser calories compared to what is being used (energy) will result in drastic weight loss.

The approach has always been the same. Low calorie meal with low amount of fat combined with aerobic exercise with the aim of increasing the amount of calories used and reducing the amount ingested, which has been summarized as eating less and moving more. You should try to understand the logic in play here, and you can think of many reasons why this approach should yield the best results, but does it really work as proposed? What were the results in the end?

There are only two incontrovertible facts to these questions:

➢ The "eat less, move more" campaign has been on for over two decades now.
➢ Since its inception over 20 years ago, the obesity rate has skyrocketed all over the world.

Looking at both facts together, we can drive out two certain inferences. First, the dietary advice is excellent, although not everyone has been following it. People tend to listen to their doctors only when it is about health-related issues. When doctors advised everyone to check their cholesterol and blood pressure level, everyone ran and checked their cholesterol and blood pressure. Somehow, people failed to listen when doctors advised to start eating less to be able to move more. At this point, the victims should be blamed, because the advice is considered to be a good one, but yet somehow, most refused to follow it.

Those who might have refused at some point would have their reasons, which might have been the inability to adjust to the new dietary plan.

"Eat less, Move More" will not work for a great percentage of people, because there is a pattern by which the body makes use of calories, and making a sharp switch to eat less and to move more will not work for those particular people who cannot adjust to the change it will bring to their body system.

How does the body use calories?

The main reason why it would be difficult for the approach "eat less, move more" to work for weight loss is that it rests on a wrong idea about how the body makes use of calories. Let us begin with the single compartment model that centres on how the body breaks down all food consumed into the simplest units (calories), and thereafter stores the calories in the single compartment for use. The normal demand for different metabolic actions prompt the body to access the compartment in order to extract calories that are used for basal metabolism, helping with the removal of toxins from the bloodstream, breathing, digestion of food, and exercise, etc.

Think of the single compartment model as a sink, and the calories like water, which with ease can flow into or out of the sink. After the body might have used the normal calories required for daily metabolic activities, the excess calories stored in this sink can still be accessed when the body requires more calories. Aerobic exercise for instance would drain a lot of calories from this sink. All calories stored in the body are treated the same way, be it stored as glucose which is used almost every second if active, or as glycogen, which is used as the intermediate, or fat, which is stored for long term usage.

This model however does not differentiate well enough, so using the two-compartment model seems more accurate and fitting. Energy is stored in two different ways in the body: either as body fat or as glycogen in the liver.

The body gets energy from three sources when food is ingested and absorbed: protein, carbohydrates in form of glucose, and fat. Two of these sources are stored in order to be used in the future - fat and glucose. Glucose is converted to glycogen and is stored in the liver, and the rest not used is stored as body fat. Initially, this was the reason why health experts recommended low-fat diets, but weight gain is not actually defined by the first destination of calories ingested. Glycogen can be seen as a refrigerator that has been designed to store food temporarily, although food can be moved in or out, but the space available for storage is limited.

Body fat on the other hand acts like a freezer designed to store food for a long time with a great capacity, although access is restricted. Energy is absorbed from ingested food and first stored as glycogen, and when the body's storage is filled up, it redirects it as body fat. Both of them (glycogen and body fat) are used for energy when food is absent, though not at the same time and not equally. The body is designed to make use of the glycogen first before switching to body fat.

According to the analogy made earlier, burning glycogen first would be easier, as it is with getting food from the fridge. In other words, if your body is going to require 400 calories of energy to go for a walk, the energy will be collected from glycogen as long as the availability is certain, not body fat.

Remember, these two energy stores are used sequentially, and not simultaneously, either your body burns sugar or burns fat, not both at once.

Chapter 5 Types of Intermittent Fasting

Intermittent fasting is the best way to improve your overall health and reach your fitness goals. For everything from giving you the required nutrition and reducing the risk of chronic diseases to weight loss and burning fat – intermittent fasting has proved its mettle in many ways. There are several types of intermittent fasts which can be implemented. We will be looking at the few popularly used and effective ones, such as:

- 6:8 method
- 5:2 method
- Eat-Stop-Eat
- Alternate-day fasting
- Warrior diet
- 16:8 Method

The 16:8 method (16 hours OFF and 8 hours ON) is also known as the daily window fasting. It is the easiest and the most popular intermittent fasting method followed by the majority. All you need to do is skip a meal! In this fasting method, you eat for 8 hours and fast for 16 hours. There are two ways of doing it:

- Skip breakfast and eat later in the day

- Or have an early dinner and don't eat anything until the next day (breakfast).

Some people do slight a bit of modification in the eating window, such as eating within one or 3 hours during the day and fast for 20 or 23 hours a day, i.e., 23:1 or 20:4 method. But when you fast for more than 20 hours, it is called the Warrior diet.

When you follow 16:8 fasting method, you eat within the 8-hour window (maybe, 11 a.m. – 7 p.m.) and then fast for the remaining 16 hours (7 p.m. until 11 a.m.). The fasting and eating window can vary depending on the individual. You can eat within a four-hour window or go for a seven-hour window, i.e., 20:4 or 17:7.

But the best choice would be to fast for 16 hours, which is inclusive of your sleeping hours. You can skip breakfast and have lunch as your first meal of the day and then finish the day with an early dinner. For instance, fast from 8 p.m. to 12 noon (16 hours – including sleep time) and have your first meal (lunch) at 12:30 p.m. and then dinner around 7 p.m. If you want, you can have snacks (fruit or veggies) around 4 p.m.

You can follow this method whenever you like – maybe twice a week or during the weekdays. You can also do it regularly for better results. When you are regular with this diet pattern, you get into the habit and your appetite also considerably reduces.

5:2 Method

This diet is the most popular intermittent fasting diet pattern as of now. It is also known as The Fast Diet. Michael Mosley, a British doctor and journalist, popularized this diet pattern.

It got its name - 5:2 diet - as you go on with your normal eating routine for five days and then restrict the calorie-intake for the remaining two days. You should only have 500-600 calories per day on those two days. You cannot call this a diet, as it is more of an eating pattern.

You don't find any restriction on what food you should eat, but it is more to do with when you should eat your food.

This is pretty easy – for five days a week, you just continue with your normal eating routine. No worries about restricting calories! You need to focus on the remaining two days of the week - the days when you should restrict your calorie consumption to 500 to 600 per day. (The math is 500 for women and 600 for men per day).

You can choose the two days as per your convenience, but the only thing to remember is you need to ensure you have a day's gap (non-fasting day) between the two days.

You can fast on Mondays and Wednesdays – 2 or 3 small meals on those two days with a check on the calories. The remaining days you can carry on with your regular food routine. However, it is important to eat the right food during the non-fasting days too – healthy, well-balanced, wholesome meals.

Eating processed food, meat, oily food, junk, etc. will not serve any purpose – as you will not be able to lose weight but on the contrary might put on more weight.

There shouldn't be too much of hogging or overeating on your non-fasting day – it should be the same quantity of food you eat normally. This dieting pattern is said to be the best to lose weight and improve your body's metabolic rate.

Eat-Stop-Eat

Eat-Stop-Eat aims to give the body a complete break from food for 24 hours. It is quite simple – you can fast once or maybe twice a week (depending on your routine). For instance, you can eat normally until 7 p.m. today and then fast until 7 p.m. the next day. You can then resume your normal eating routine (try sticking to the healthy and wholesome diet). You can repeat the fast after several days (after, maybe, two or three weeks).

One important thing to remember is - do not exceed two fasts in one week! Fasting once in a week should be more than enough, but if you feel you can manage with two, you can still go ahead!

You need to ensure your body is hydrated during your fasting days. You can have water, black coffee and herbal tea. In case you feel hungry, you can have a smoothie or cold-pressed fresh juice (without sugar or sweetener).

Similarly, when you break your fast, you can eat normally but ensure you don't indulge in overeating, as that would ruin the benefits of the fast. It is good to include a lot of vegetables, spices and fruit in your diet during your non-fasting days.

If you are following the Eat-Stop-Eat diet pattern to your regular routine, you can combine a consistent workout routine for your non-fasting days. But ensure you don't exercise on your fasting days as you might end up over-exerting your body muscles. This diet might cause headaches in some people.

Pregnant women, nursing mothers, people with diabetes or people with eating disorders should not observe this diet. You will need a good amount of self-control and should be able to decide which food will be good for you.

Alternate-day Fasting

Alternate day fasting or ADF is another type of intermittent fasting which works well for longevity and weight loss. The rules are quite simple – you fast alternate days, no calorie-intake should be present during your fast days, and you can eat normally during your eating days.

You can have only water during your fast days or can consume water and other fluids (black coffee, herbal tea, fresh juices, etc.), but none of the fluids should have sugar or sweetener added to them.

This fasting method has numerous benefits but only when it is done the right way. A healthy choice of food is more important. Combining exercise with your diet plan will be more effective towards your weight-loss goal as well as for your overall health. Ensure you don't eat processed food, as it might do no good to your health. Your food plate must have a combination of vegetables, fruit, spices and wholesome meal.

Most people will find this intermittent fasting method an easier choice, but some may find it difficult. People who eat more than three meals in a day might find it difficult. There are some who get irritated when they miss a meal – this pattern will not work for them either.

But again, it is fine! Each of us has our own individuality – the body metabolism, dietary choices, preferences and activity levels will be different.

The Warrior Diet

The Warrior diet is a combination of exercise and fasting. You will need to follow your gut feeling when it comes to choosing the right diet. Avoid getting tempted by processed food or junk food. Don't get too rigid with the types of macronutrients and calories that need to be consumed during the eating window. Instead, as the name implies, eat like a warrior! Our prehistoric warriors had little food during the day and had their meal at night, i.e., little food in the day and more food at night.

The Warrior diet is more to do with vigorous exercising (even during the fasting days) and controlled food-intake. You will need to exercise when your stomach is completely empty (preferably as soon as you wake up). You will have only one meal in a day. If you can adapt to this type of intermittent fasting, you will be able to burn more fat (into energy) and will get a lean physique without the need to count your calories.

Your exercise routine should be total body strength training – squats, pushups, pull-ups, high jumps, skipping and presses. You can also include high-intensity cardio exercises, such as frog jumps or sprints, in between these sessions. These sessions can last for between 20 and 45 minutes.

Since you can have only one meal in a day, you might take time to get adapted to this routine. You might feel weak or dizzy initially. Don't push it too hard! First, introduce your body to the diet routine gradually – maybe skip breakfast twice a week and eat your lunch and dinner as usual. Continue this for few weeks, then slowly skip two meals and get your body accustomed to the routine. Once your body is ready, get into the full-on warrior diet mode. Don't under-eat, eat normally during your non-fasting days. Include more whole, raw foods to enable your digestive enzymes to help you.

Since it is only one meal with a strong exercise regimen, you need to keep your body hydrated. Ensure you drink a lot of water and consume fluids like herbal tea, black coffee, fresh juice (cold-pressed) with no sugar or sweetener. You can also have green smoothies (without butter or cream). When you focus on drinking cold-pressed juices (from the whole food) or whole raw food, you are helping your body to reload, as these foods are full of enzymes.

Make sure you have a healthy organic, wholesome meal during your eating window. Add more vegetables, spices, greens and fruit to your plate. Drink enough water after your meal.

This diet might not be suitable for the general public as it might not fit into their daily lifestyles, work routines, body capacities, etc. Moreover, it is quite difficult to get all the required nutrients your body needs in just one meal every day.

Sometimes, this diet can leave you so hungry that you indulge in pigging the food, which will result in overeating. And this is definitely not going to help you lose weight. Similarly, not many people will be okay with exercising (especially strength training) on an empty stomach. They might feel dizzy and have a nauseous feeling.

It is, therefore, better to check with your physician before choosing this fasting method – or any method for that matter.

Listen to your body and choose the style that will best suit your routine. It should bring the best in your body's health making you feel energetic and lighter.

Chapter 6 Tips for Intermittent Fasting

Getting started with intermittent fasting can take some time. You will have to change some of the eating patterns that you are used to, but it can be effective for you in so many ways. You will see that it is easier to lose weight, improve your energy, burn body fat, get more done, and protect against diseases such as diabetes, cancer, and dementia.

Although intermittent fasting is easier than most other diet plans out there, it still takes some work. Some of the things to keep in mind to get the most out of your intermittent fast are:

Drink plenty of water: Water keeps you hydrated and makes you feel fuller when you are on your fast. Being in a fasted state also acts as a diuretic, which means that your body will naturally expel water at a faster rate than you are used to. What it all boils down to is that you are going to want to aim to consume a gallon of water a day for the best results.

Drink tea and coffee: When you are feeling hungry, you may find that it's helpful to drink tea or coffee to keep down your appetite. Caffeine is a natural appetite suppressant. Just try not to consume any caffeine too close to bedtime (at least 3 hours), or you may have trouble falling asleep.

Keep yourself busy: You may find that are more productive on an empty stomach. If you are keeping yourself busy, not only will you get more done, but you'll be able to distract yourself from the hunger. If you don't find productive ways to fill your time, especially at first, then you will find that the hours you are fasting seem to stretch out into days. Don't make things harder on yourself than they need to be. When it comes to the early days of your new eating habit, make sure your days are packed full of activities.

Make it flexible: There are so many options that come with intermittent fasting. You do not have to go with one option because everyone else is. You can mix and match and create the schedule that works for you. Intermittent fasting is all about having the freedom to do it the way that you want.

Try it for at least a month: You need at least three to four weeks to determine if the intermittent fast is right for you. If you don't do it for this long, then you are not giving the body the time it needs to adapt, and you are not giving it a fair shot. Try it out for at least this amount of time to see if it's the right choice for you.

Experiment with fasting methods: What works for one person may not work for you. If you find that certain fasting times are better or that a particular version of intermittent fasting is more effective, then choose those. It's all experimenting to see what feels right for you.

Delay your breakfast slowly: One thing that works well for a lot of people is to slowly delay their breakfast. By gradually pushing back your breakfast time an hour every week or so, you will eventually get yourself into an intermittent fast without it being too difficult. For instance, if you usually eat breakfast at 8 am, wait until 8:30 am to eat your breakfast for the first week. Then push your breakfast back to 9 am in week 2. Continue this process until your first meal occurs around noon.

Drink water in the morning: Often the reason that you feel so hungry in the morning is that you have gone all night without eating. A good habit to start is to drink a glass of water right when you wake up in the morning.

Add weights: If you are trying to lose weight and tone up, it makes sense to add some weight training to your routine. While you won't want to mix things up too much when you are first getting started, once your body has adapted to an intermittent fasting lifestyle, there is no reason you shouldn't take things up a notch. You will be surprised what your body can handle. If you take things slowly, eventually you should be able to handle a full-intensity workout without feeling too drained to function when you are finished.

Live it up: With intermittent fasting, you need to realize that you can live it up on occasion. You can have fun as long as you ensure it all balances out in the end. While the average diet is all about the foods that you aren't allowed to eat, an intermittent fasting lifestyle accounts for the fact that sometimes you can't plan your meals. This means that as long as you get your fasting period in, there is no reason you can't move your hours around, as long as you don't do so constantly. What's more, there is no reason you can't indulge now and then, as long as one delicious and decadent dessert doesn't end up turning into seven or eight.

Get out of the house: There is a lot of temptation in your home. Therefore, it is better to get out of the house, so you don't eat all of that food. Even if you have kids around, think of an activity you all can do to keep yourselves occupied.

Eat more protein and healthy fat: Eating additional protein with each meal makes it easier to control your appetite and build up your muscles. Eating more healthy fat will give you extra energy and help you feel fuller longer as well. Thanks to the insidious advancement of the Standard American Diet, a vast majority of those in the Western world eat far too many carbohydrates and not nearly enough protein or healthy fat. To rectify this problem, start considering the macros of the foods you eat. Also, ensure that when you are in an eating window you fill your plate with foods that will make sticking it out to the next window as easy as possible.

Avoid the bad stuff: You need to make sure that you are not using it as an excuse to eat junk food all the time. Make sure to stick with a well-balanced diet so that you provide your body with enough nutrition, even if you choose to go on a fast. It is important to keep in mind that a big part of intermittent fasting is building up a calorie deficit by the end of the week to support additional weight loss. As such, if you fill your body full of high-calorie junk food when you do enter an eating window, what you are really doing is undoing all of your hard work. Making healthy choices at all times will improve the overall effectiveness of your weight loss efforts, guaranteed.

As you can see, there are a lot of different things you can do to get the most out of intermittent fasting. This doesn't mean you should expect constant weight loss, however, regardless of how strict your fasting might be. While you will likely see weight loss at first as your body adapts to fewer calories in its system; this will likely start and stop throughout your time fasting. The effects are especially noticeable after the first few weeks of the transition as your body tries to hold on to everything it has until it can figure out what is going on. Once it gets with the program, however, things should proceed as expected.

Every diet is going to have periods of weight loss plateau. That is simply a part of weight loss that cannot be mitigated. As long as you stay consistent, weight loss will eventually resume. The worst thing you can do is to try and change things up to get weight loss back on track as that will only make it more difficult for your body to start losing weight again. Instead, if you stay the course and keep up the good work, you will start seeing results again before you know it.

Chapter 7 Intermittent Fast FAQs

There are a lot of questions that you may have with intermittent fasting. You want to make sure that you are doing it the right way and that you will be able to get all the benefits that are promised with this diet plan. This chapter will take some time to explore more about intermittent fasting and what you need to know to get it to work for you.

Is there anyone who shouldn't fast?

For the most part, intermittent fasting is safe for most people to do. It's an effective diet plan that focuses on healthy eating and getting the essential calories and nutrition that your body needs while restricting the windows that you're allowed to eat.

With that said, some people should not go on an intermittent fast. This is mostly because there is concern that they will not be able to get the nutrition that they need. If you're considered underweight, you should not go on this kind of fast. If you're pregnant or breastfeeding, you need to take in nutrients throughout the day to support your child, so intermittent fasting is not the option for you.

In addition, there are times when you are allowed to fast, but you may want to make sure that you have some supervision from your doctor. First, if you have diabetes, either type 1 or type 2, you will need to do this with the help of your doctor. Some medications don't work well with these fasts so you will need to be careful. In addition, if you have high uric acid or gout, you may need to be careful about going on an intermittent fast.

Will I go into starvation mode if I am fasting?

There are a lot of myths about fasting. These myths are repeated so often that sometimes they are seen as truths. Some of the fasting myths that you may know about include:

➢ Fasting makes you starve
➢ Fasting will you feel hungry
➢ Fasting will make you overeat when the fast is over
➢ Fasting will make you lose muscle tone

These have been disproven many times over. Instead of the body going into starvation mode, the body will start burning up the extra fat stored inside. This will help you to get rid of that stubborn belly fat and will help you become healthier, especially if you have been overeating for a long time.

Over a year, you consume about 1000 meals and over 60 years, you will eat about 60,000 meals. To say that skipping three meals during this time will cause a lot of harm is kind of silly.

The breakdown of muscle tissue only occurs at low levels of body fat, and if you are at that point, then you shouldn't go on a fast. However, most people will not have this issue. Our bodies are actually evolved to handle periods of starvation and will be able to effectively deal with it.

What are some side effects of going on a fast?

There are a few side effects that you can deal with when you are on a fast. These are usually pretty simple, and they will go away after your body adjusts to the diet and you get familiar with eating habits that work well. Some of the side effects that you may experience include:

Constipation: This is a common side effect. If you're experiencing constipation, using some laxatives can to help to alleviate the pain or discomfort.

Headaches: Some people experience headaches when they get started on a fast, but these will disappear within a few days. A good way to deal with this is to eat some extra salt each day.

Mineral water: If you are dealing with your stomach gurgling, then it is a good idea to use mineral water.

Other side effects: You may also deal with issues such as muscle cramps, dizziness, and heartburn. Adjusting your diet and waiting a few days will help to alleviate any discomfort.

How do I manage hunger?

The most important thing to realize is that this hunger will pass. Most people worry that the hunger will keep growing until it is intolerable, but this usually isn't the case. Hunger comes in waves. Ignoring it and drinking some water, tea, or coffee will help you to cope with the hunger pains.

During your extended fast, you might notice that the hunger will increase into the second day. After you get past that time, you will see that it recedes, with many people reporting that they have a complete loss of hunger by day 3 or 4. At this time, your body is powered by fat. This means that the body is eating its own fat for breakfast, lunch, and dinner, so you are no longer feeling so hungry. So, if you can last a few days on the intermittent fast, the hunger pains will go away, and it will be easier to deal with.

It is important to keep in mind that when you are first starting out your body is likely to struggle with fasting because it is used to have ready access to fuel all the time. Most of us are used to eating, even when we are not hungry, and the body will fight against your new habit with extreme hunger pains in an effort to get back on track. However, whether you go with the 16/8 fast, the 5:2 fast, or the alternate day fast, the truth of the matter is that you are not putting your body through anything it cannot handle. As such, as long as you stay the course, things will likely settle down in about a week or so once your body realizes that it is not, in fact, starving.

In order to make the transition as manageable as possible, the first thing you are going to want to do is to add more caffeine to your diet. While not acceptable in the long-term, this is a great way to keep the worst of the hunger pains away when they are at their sharpest. Additionally, you will want to ensure that your schedule is full during this time as the more activity your mind has to focus on, the faster time will fly. Finally, if you are already committed to an exercise plan, then you will want to ensure that you exercise right before you break your fast so that your body will get the fuel it needs to make the most of your efforts.

Will my fasting burn muscle?

This is a common misconception that a lot of people deal with when they are considering an intermittent fast. During the fasting periods, the body is first going to break down the glycogen into glucose so that it can be used for energy. After the glucose is all gone, the body will increase how much fat it's breaking down and use that for energy. Excess amino acids, which are the building blocks of protein, can also be used for energy. However, the body is not going to use its own muscle as fuel unless you're not eating for weeks on end.

Fasting is a practice that has been done for thousands of years. It's safe and effective, and unless you go for weeks without eating (and none of the intermittent fasting options ask you to fast for more than 24 hours), there is no reason to worry about losing excess muscle.

How do I break the fast?

Breaking the fast is one of the hardest parts of this diet and is likely the true test of whether or not you will be able to sustain it in the long-term. When you break your fast it is important to do so in moderation for multiple reasons. First, it is important to not add too much to your system all at once as this can put stress on your body and damage your stomach and intestines if repeated too often. Additionally, if you allow yourself to gorge when your resolve is at its weakest then you are far more likely to overeat and undue all the hard work you have done by fasting in the first place.

The best way to ensure that this does not happen is to plan ahead. Prepare the meal while you are waiting for the fast to end and ensure that it has very clearly defined portions. A hearty omelet is a good choice as you can fill it full of healthy, filling items and you can't easily go back for seconds. Meanwhile, a full pot of oatmeal is a poor choice as you could easily go through it without thinking twice.

Can women fast?

Yes, women can fast. The only exception to this rule is if you're underweight, pregnant, or breastfeeding. This is because you need those extra nutrients and should not go so long without eating in these situations. Other than that, it is perfectly fine for women to fast. In addition, the average weight loss with fasting is the same for men and women so it can be effective for both genders.

Tips for intermittent fasting

Getting started with intermittent fasting can be a challenge at times. To summarize, tips you can follow include:

- Drink lots of water
- Stay busy
- Drink coffee or tea to suppress hunger
- Find a good support group who can help you
- Ride out the hunger waves because they will go away
- Try to go on a low-carb diet. This will help you with reducing hunger and can make fasting easier. It can also help out with more weight loss.
- Give it a month
- Break a fast gently
- Do not binge when you are done with fasting

Chapter 8 : Myths Concerning Intermittent Fasting

Myth 1: Starvation Mode

Many people believe that by eating in a caloric deficit or fasting regularly will put your body into starvation mode. Meaning that this will cause your body to adapt by shutting down your metabolic rate, making you burn fewer calories. But most of the time people cut their calories so low at the beginning it causes the body to shift gears to conserve energy for the person to perform regular daily tasks. To preserve energy the body begins searching for anything to hold onto. Which the first target is your muscle and not the fat you are trying to eliminate.

Your body is a piece of art and works more efficiently when using the calories, you consume than wasting them. So, by implementing intermittent fasting, you will not have to cut your calories so low as science has proved that fasting can increase your metabolic rate by up to 14%. Which will allow you to save your muscle and help you burn more fat.

Myth 2: Intermittent Fasting causes binge eating

Binge eating may come to mind when thinking about intermittent fasting or any kind of fasting. If you have ever done any kind of fasting (Personal, physical, spiritual) then you know that at the end of your fasting window you experienced extreme cravings. So many people automatically link binge eating with "IF" when thinking of this. But there have been many studies on the two and how they are related.

One study showed that a group of people who fasted an entire day (24hrs) overate the next day by an average of 500 calories. Well, scientifically it is proven that the average person burns 2,000 calories a day. If that is so, then that would place the person from the group in a 1500 caloric deficit in only 48hrs since the 24hr fast the day before!

This study proves that overeating is a factor that has no correlation to intermittent fasting.

Myth3: Skipping Breakfast

"Breakfast is the most important meal of the day" is a term that we have all heard before. Since being a small child, our parents and guardians have instilled in us that eating breakfast will set off our day in a positive way. We have been told that skipping breakfast causes weakness, fatigue, low concentration levels, and makes your body crave bad foods. Several scientific studies have shown that this is not the case concerning energy levels and only a myth.

Other studies done link skipping breakfast to obesity and low performance rates in schools. But these studies did not consider the timing it takes for your body to get accustomed to this new tool or lifestyle. You can't just start skipping breakfast then began measuring your performance or energy levels. You can't start intermittent fasting and expect not to be hungry after the first fast. You should be patient, start slowly and allow your body to adjust to this new eating styles.

Myth 4: 6 small meals a day for metabolic increase

Eating small but frequent meals throughout the day will raise your metabolic rate is true! But it is not the end of all tools and tricks to burn more calories. Around 10% of the calories we eat are burned off during digestion which is called the thermic effect of food or

TEF. But this effect is caused by how many calories we consume not by how many meals we eat.

Let's say a person ate 6 small meals, measuring 500 calories each then the next day ate 3 meals totaling 1,000 calories each. On both days the person ate 3,000 calories and burned the same 10% of the total calories. Measuring about 300 calories burned on both days. So as you see this myth does not trump the effects of intermittent fasting.

There are many myths and false information on and off the internet. Be sure to diligently search for truth and slow to judge when researching any topic.

Conclusion

So, there you have it — intermittent fasting in a nutshell. Despite what you may think about not eating for so many hours, it will not kill you and, trust me, you will not feel all that hungry either. The real trick is to make sure that you eat properly and eat the right foods during your feeding window and, that you drink plenty of fluids, especially water.

Intermittent fasting has so many benefits and very few, if any downsides. A lot of people have gotten fantastic results with some of the intermittent fasting methods listed in this book. Still, it really will not work for everyone so do not feel put out if it doesn't work for you. It may be that you are on the wrong protocol so try another one. If you are fasting for 24 hours twice a week, give the 16/8 a go and fast for 16 hours every day. Even just twelve to fourteen hours or so of fasting can be beneficial — skip breakfast, or dinner, if you cannot bring yourself to skip both or find that doing so does not work for you personally. It is easier if you make sure that your fasting period covers your sleeping time. If you work nights, change your feeding period to the nighttime and your fasting period to the day, when you are sleeping. Also, do not forget that the effect of intermittent fasting will be rendered pointless if you binge on junk food during eating periods. Whether fasting or not, the quality of your food is absolutely essential.

One thing I must stress is this — do consult with a physician before you start any intermittent fasting protocol. Intermittent fasting is completely safe for the vast majority of people, but there are some factors that could encourage your physician to recommend against it. Certain medical conditions and certain medications prohibit fasting and you may end up feeling worse or your medications may not work for you. Additionally, if you are very thin, especially if that is due to an eating disorder or if you are prone to weakness and fainting, you may need to gain some weight or otherwise ensure your previous conditions are deemed medically safe before you begin. Even when you consult a physician while on the diet, you may find that there are no changes that have been made to your body. Our bodies all change at different rates. Some of us can lose weight easily and some of us struggle more than others to gain muscle mass. You might find one of your desired results not appearing as quickly as you thought (and hoped) that it would when you began your fast. It is during this time that you keep yourself motivated since quitting the diet will never help you in any way! Good luck!

Thank you again for downloading this book.

I hope this book was able to help you to answer all questions pertaining intermittent fasting.

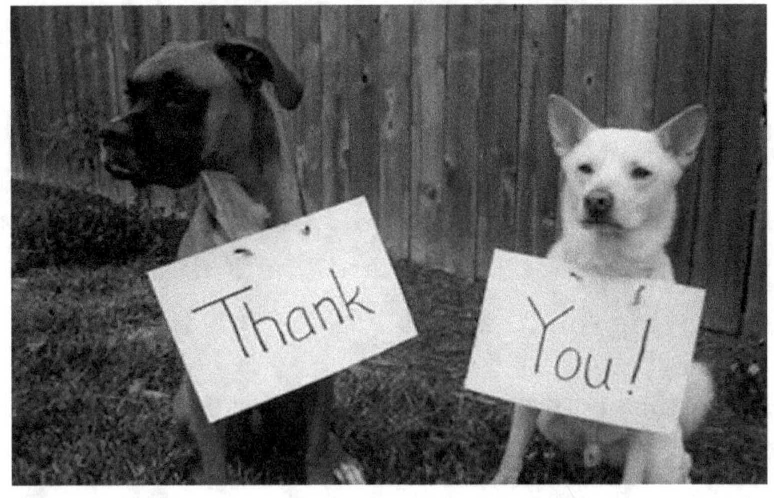

Finally, if you enjoyed this book, then I'd like to ask you for a favor, would you be kind enough to leave a review for this book on Amazon? It'd be greatly appreciated!

Click here to leave a review for this book on Amazon!

Thank you and good luck!

Check Out My Other Books

Below you'll find some of my other popular books that are popular on Amazon and Kindle as well. Simply click on the links below to check them out. Alternatively, you can visit our author page on Amazon to see other work done by Achievement Pyramid.

https://www.amazon.com/dp/B07C189PB3 - **Weight Loss: Igniting Your Weight Loss Motivation: Five Proven Steps to Get You Back On Track**

https://www.amazon.com/dp/B07D5H25S5 - **Weight Loss: The Fundamental Guide to Achieving the Right Body Size You Want**

If the links do not work, for whatever reason, you can simply search for these titles on the Amazon website to find them.

Us: Subscribe To The Pyramid Building Toolkit

When you subscribe to Achievement Pyramid via email, you will get our newsletter and emails about our upcoming books. All you have to do is enter your email address to the right to get instant access.

This will help you get more out of your life – to be able to reach your goals, have more motivation, be at your best, and live the life you've always dreamed of. We are making new books all the time as well, which you will be notified of as a subscriber. **These will help you live life to the fullest!**

Click here for the Pyramid Building Toolkit.

Or you can access it here: http://eepurl.com/dv48LX